DRUGS AND DEPRESSION

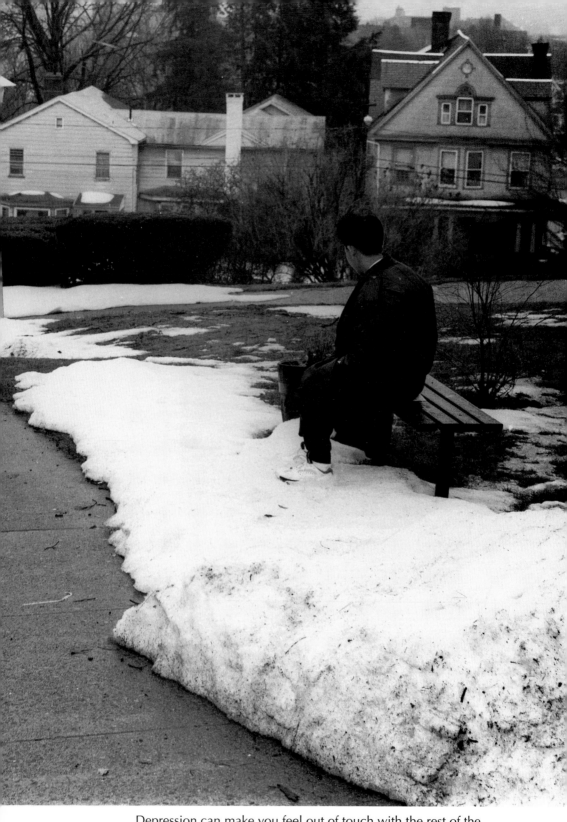

Depression can make you feel out of touch with the rest of the world.

DRUGS AND DEPRESSION

Beth Wilkinson

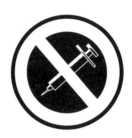

THE ROSEN PUBLISHING GROUP, INC.

NEW YORK

Published in 1994, 1999 by The Rosen Publishing Group, Inc.
29 East 21st Street, New York, NY 10010

Library of Congress Cataloging-in-Publication Data

Wilkinson, Beth
   Drugs and depression / by Beth Wilkinson.
     p. cm. —(The Drug abuse prevention library)
   Includes bibliographical references and index.
   ISBN 0-8239-3004-1
    1. Teenagers—Substance use—Juvenile literature. 2. Depression in adolescence—Juvenile literature. 3. Substance abuse—Juvenile literature. [1. Depression, Mental. 2. Drug abuse.] I. Title. II. Series.
RJ506.D78W55 1993
616.86'00835—dc20
                                    93-36366
                                         CIP
                                       AC

Manufactured in the United States of America

Contents

Introduction

*D*epression can last a few minutes or it can last a lifetime. The feeling can be mild or miserable. Most people are able to overcome short periods of being "down" and get on with their lives.

Depression can also be an unhealthy sadness accompanied by fatigue, headache, and bizarre behavior. This type of depression may be caused by a biochemical instability. That means an imbalance of the chemicals called neurotransmitter molecules that ordinarily guide and organize activity in the brain.

Often, in our society, people look for quick fixes for problems and depression. Many people mistakenly believe that drugs are a solution or that drugs will relieve their bad feelings. Trying to hide drug use, trying to get money to buy drugs, and trying to stay in school can actually *cause* worry and depression. Some claim that they can use drugs and alcohol with moderation. They say "no problem"; they think they can handle it. For a while it may seem to work, but experimenting with drugs is like waiting for a bomb to go off. When it explodes, it scatters pieces of broken families, sick bodies, and low self-esteem under an even greater cloud of emptiness, sadness, and pain.

In fact, if a close family member was an alcoholic, an experimenting teen is more likely at risk. Also, because their bodies are still developing, young people become addicted easily.

The first step for the person caught in the trap of drugs and depression is to admit that something is wrong. Next, he or she needs to get help. Trained school counselors and social workers are ready to assist young people. Many teachers are also willing to talk with their students. Most communities provide support, counseling, and care for troubled people of all ages. If you are trying to get off drugs and trying to fight depression at the same time, then you need help. Talk to someone you trust. Get the help you need. (See the Help List at the back of this book.) Taking control of your life may be the best "high" you ever have.

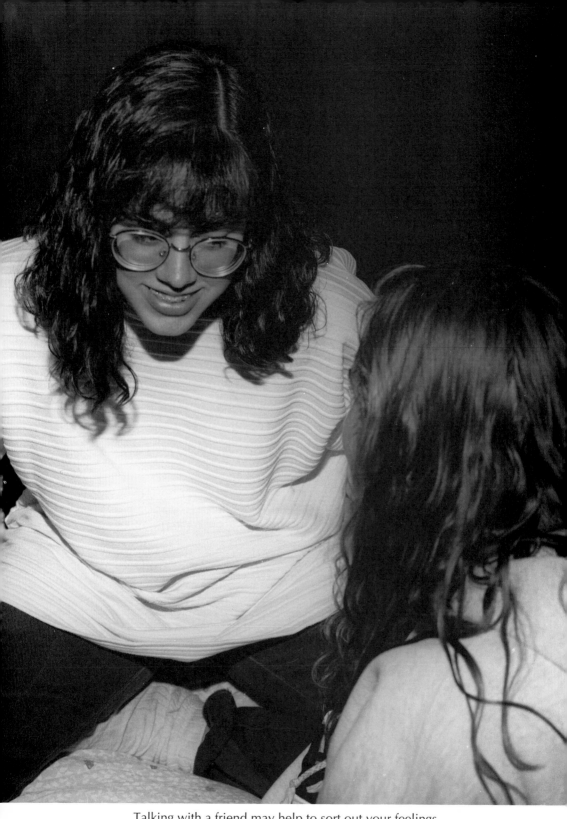

Talking with a friend may help to sort out your feelings.

CHAPTER 1

When Stress and Anxiety Hit Hard

*E*very year, 17.6 million Americans, almost 10 percent of the U.S. population, suffer from a depressive illness. Depression can interfere with a person's normal functioning and can cause much anguish. The saddest fact about depression is that most sufferers do not seek help. With proper treatment, full recovery is possible.

Depression involves your body and mind. It varies from mild symptoms to serious mental illness. It affects the way you eat and sleep, the way you feel about yourself and the world around you. It can be caused by a serious loss or death, a chronic illness, a difficult relationship, financial problems, job or school difficulties, or a disappointment or rejection.

10 In fact any unwelcome change can trigger a depressive episode.

Most teenagers experience feelings of depression. Becoming independent is not easy. When things go wrong, teenagers often look for easy solutions or a way to escape. Some turn to drugs. Drugs are not a solution. When the drug wears off, people become even more depressed, and the problems remain.

Types of Depression

Depression and depressive disorders come in different forms. Three of the most common types of depression are:

- *Major depression*—the sufferer has a combination of symptoms that interfere with day-to-day functioning. These painful episodes can occur once, twice, or even several times in a lifetime.
- *Dysthymia*—a less severe type of depression involving long-term symptoms that keep you from operating at "full steam" or from feeling good.
- *Bipolar disorder*—formerly called manic depression. It is generally caused by a biochemical imbalance in the brain, and it can be controlled with appropriate medicines. A person

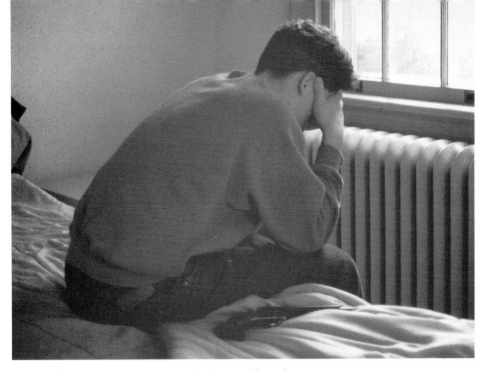

Severe depression can cause confusion and hopelessness. Unfortunately, some teens think suicide is the only way out.

with a bipolar disorder often has up-and-down feelings called mood swings. He or she goes from experiencing very high highs (mania) to very low lows (depression). These mood swings may happen very quickly, but most often they are gradual. Mania often affects judgment and social behavior in ways that can cause embarrassment. A person experiencing mania may make unwise decisions.

Symptoms of Depression and Mania

Not everyone who is depressed or manic experiences each of the symptoms below. Some people experience a few symptoms, while other people may experience many.

12 Depression
- Constant sad, anxious mood
- Feelings of hopelessness or negativity
- Feelings of guilt or worthlessness
- Loss of interest in hobbies and activities
- Insomnia (sleeplessness), early-morning awakening, or oversleeping
- Change in appetite; fasting or over-eating; weight loss or weight gain
- Decreased energy or being "slowed down"
- Difficulty concentrating, remember-ing things, or making decisions
- Self-mutilation
- Thoughts of death or suicide; suicide attempts

Mania
- Inappropriate joy or enthusiasm
- Inappropriate irritability
- Inability to sleep
- Inflated notions and ideas
- Increased talking
- Disconnected and racing thoughts
- Poor judgment
- Inappropriate social behavior

Related Disorders
Depression and anxiety often go together. When people cannot control events, they

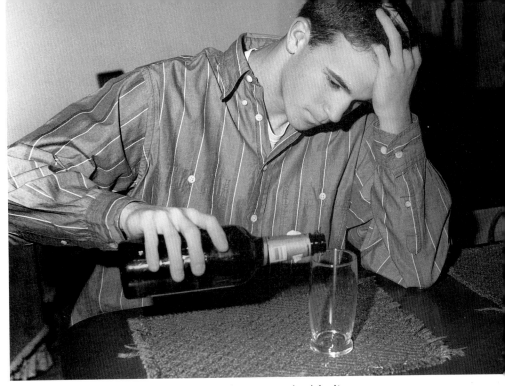

Drinking does not solve problems. It only worsens bad feelings and prolongs depression.

may become hopeless, negative, and despairing. There are many types and symptoms of anxiety disorders.

Panic attacks occur when the body has magnified physical responses to situations in which there is no danger present. Panic is the body's way of preparing a person to flee or fight when encountering a threat. Fear and panic are normal reactions to danger. They set off a chain reaction in the body by activating the biological and chemical regulators of breathing, digestion, and temperature. When you experience a panic attack, adrenaline is released into your body, but, since there is no danger to contend with,

14 the body cannot get rid of the adrenaline for what seems like a very long time. People who have had panic attacks are usually afraid of having further attacks. The feeling of being out of control— pounding heart, hyperventilating, sweating, and numbness—is so overwhelming that they will do almost anything to avoid feeling that way again.

Generalized Anxiety Disorder happens when a person experiences excessive worry, usually for at least six months, for no apparent reason. Muscle tension evidenced by trembling, twitching, fatigue, and restlessness is one of the common symptoms. There may be sweating and hot flashes or chills. Even in moments of relaxation, a person with a generalized anxiety disorder may feel irritable or keyed-up or may have difficulty concentrating.

Specific Phobias are unreasonable fears of a particular object or event. People are phobic about various things. Many people are afraid of heights. They fear falling, or they feel impelled to jump. Others are afraid of snakes, spiders, dogs, strangers, closed-in spaces, dentists, or even water. When people are afraid of certain things, we say they are suffering from specific phobias. These people are not truly phobic, however, until they start avoiding, or wanting to avoid, the thing that frightens them.

Often, specific phobias happen because of bad experiences that left a painful emotional scar. People injured in car accidents are sometimes phobic about driving.

Many people are uncomfortable around certain things. This does not mean that they have a phobia. A fear is not a phobia unless you have to change your life in order to cope with the fear.

Social Phobias differ from specific phobias in that the real fear is of embarassing yourself. The most common social phobia is the fear of speaking in public. Fear of choking while eating in public is the second most common fear. People may be afraid of using the bathroom in public, eating in public, or even using the telephone in public. People who suffer from social phobias usually fear being observed, thinking that others are laughing at them or finding fault with them. They start avoiding places where they may start to experiencing these types of feelings.

16 | ***Posttraumatic Stress Disorder*** is another form of anxiety disorder. It occurs when someone re-experiences a severely frightening or disturbing event, bringing back the intense anxiety he or she felt when the event actually happened. It is triggered by memories, nightmares, flashbacks, or other reminders of the original incident. Rape and sexual abuse victims, disaster survivors, and soldiers have all reported this disorder. Often, posttraumatic stress disorder includes an insensitivity or numbness to people and events that remind the victim of the painful experience.

Obsessive-Compulsive Disorder means having persistent, distressing thoughts and repeating certain behaviors or acts (such as praying, or counting) to get rid of those thoughts. Many people think about an embarrassing experience over and over, or spend far too much time writing and rewriting a letter. But when such behavior interferes with their daily routine, or when not doing something exactly the same way each time causes them terrible anxiety, it may be considered an obsessive-compulsive disorder. Obsessive-compulsive disorder has two distinct parts: obsessions and compulsions.

Obsessions are unwanted, uncontrollable, or inappropriate thoughts. Constantly thinking of hitting someone over the head with a baseball bat is an obsessive thought. Compulsions then develop as a response to obsessions. Repeating certain physical or mental tasks helps to relieve the anxiety caused by the obsession. Everyone has inappropriate thoughts from time to time, and everyone has routines, but someone is said to have an obsessive-compulsive disorder when a routine interferes with the rest of his or her life.

The most common routine is "checking." Some people constantly check to see if they have turned off the stove or turned out the lights. But instead of checking once or twice, they may check thirty times. Other people have a compulsion to touch things or have rituals about getting dressed.

Emile's Morning Routine

In the morning before he goes to school, Emile has to get up from his bed on the left side. He then has to put on his slippers, left foot first. When he walks to the bathroom to take a twelve-minute shower, he must hold his left hand behind his back. This may seem funny, but Emile is not joking when he follows this routine. If for some reason he can take

18 *only an eleven-minute shower, or if he can't find his slippers, Emile becomes very upset.*

Failure to perform such rituals brings on feelings of terrible anxiety in many people. They believe that harm will come to a loved one if they don't perform their ritual. Often, obsessions and compulsions are very closely related. Someone who fears doing something sinful may pray compulsively, and someone who is obsessed with germs and contamination may compulsively wash his or her hands.

Ordinary anxiety is felt by everyone at some time. A shy teenager who doesn't want to give a speech in front of the whole class does not necessarily have a social phobia. The little girl who worries that her father will die during a complicated surgery and then prays for him doesn't necessarily have obsessive-compulsive disorder. In the face of danger, panic is normal. Anxiety is also normal. It tells us to take a look at the things that produce stress in our lives. Only when the symptoms of panic and anxiety become so disruptive that we cannot continue our daily lives do we have a disorder that needs to be treated.

CHAPTER 2

Mixing Drugs with Depression

*T*o understand how drugs and depression go hand in hand, it is first necessary to explore the reasons why teens might turn to drugs when they are feeling depressed. Then we will explore the types, uses, and effects of drugs, and how they affect depression.

A Difficult Time

Being a teen means trying new things and deciding what you like. You want to act like an adult and make your own decisions. Perhaps people around you are experimenting with drugs and it seems like a cool thing to do. Maybe you think that experimenting with drugs will help you make new friends. It is common to want to fit in with your friends at school.

20 However, it is dangerous to use a drug you don't know anything about just because you are curious.

Other teens use drugs to cope with the pressures of adolescence. Many teens who feel depressed or anxious also turn to drugs to forget their problems, to feel happy, or just to stop feeling altogther. But taking depressants ("downers") to numb bad feelings actually increases the symptoms of depression. Taking stimulants ("uppers") to battle low energy and loss of interest makes depression worse after you "come down" from a high. In short, taking drugs does not make problems or depression disappear. It only creates more problems.

The Wrong Kind of Drug

Teens who experience depression or anxiety may turn to using drugs or other substances in order to change their mood and seek relief from the pain of depression. Many drugs used in this way are not only highly addictive, but they actually worsen the symptoms of depression and anxiety. In many instances, brain damage, respiratory damage, heart failure, seizures, and death are the direct result of attempts to self-medicate. There are also indirect re-

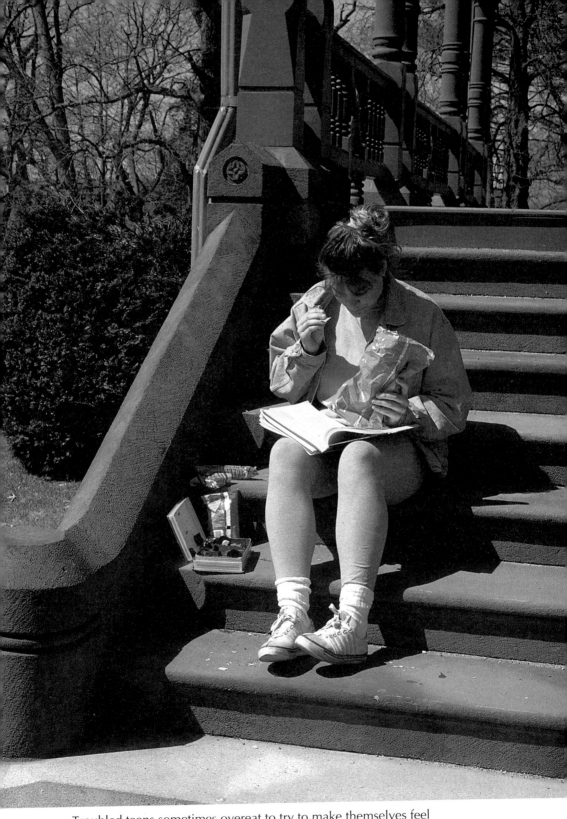

Troubled teens sometimes overeat to try to make themselves feel good.

22 | sults. Most of these drugs and substances are illegal for teenagers to possess and sell, and there are legal consequences if they are caught.

Depressants. Depressants slow down the user's mind and body, creating a feeling of relaxation and reduced anxiety. Some of the most popular depressants among young people are: barbiturates or "downers" (pills such as Seconal, Nembutal, or Quaalude), heroin and China White (a cheaper and more dangerous form of heroin), alcohol, and the nightclub favorite Special K.

Depressants are highly addictive and difficult to quit using. The addicted user has a constant craving for more drugs and a need to avoid the crash that brings on painful cramps, sweats, and chills.

Heroin users can contract HIV (the virus that causes AIDS) by sharing needles with someone who is already infected.

Stimulants. Stimulants such as cocaine and crack speed up the user's mind and body, creating a feeling of increased energy and alertness. People use them because of the brief, intense feeling of power the drug can create. This euphoria (an intense feeling of pleasure) lasts only a short time. The crash (let-down) that follows is long, leaving the user depressed, drowsy, and

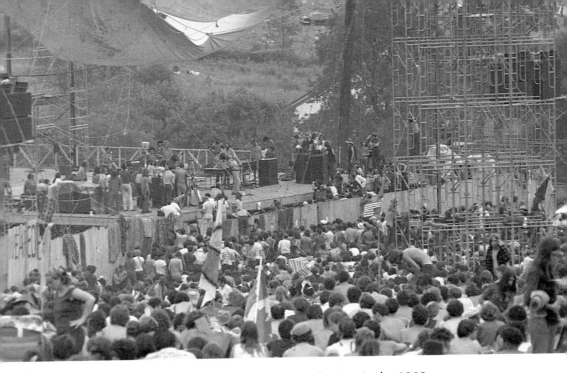

Woodstock was one of the largest peace gatherings in the 1960s. Recreational use of drugs was popular at that time.

moody. The user's craving is never satisfied. He or she constantly needs more drugs to get over the powerful depression that follows the crash. If one is already depressed before taking such drugs, the rush of negative feelings can be terrifying. Stimulants are very addictive and can cause severe paranoia and loss of self-control.

Caffeine, nicotine, and alcohol are stimulants too. Caffeine is found in coffee, tea, many soft drinks, and even in chocolate and some flavors of ice cream. Too much caffeine can be harmful, causing headaches, nervousness, and lack of sleep. Nicotine is an addictive substance found in cigarettes, cigars, pipe tobacco, and snuff.

Hallucinogens. Hallucinogens, such

24 as marijuana, hashish, LSD (acid), peyote, magic mushrooms, mescaline, PCP (angel dust), and Ecstasy, cause the user to see, hear, and feel differently. They produce feelings of extreme happiness. Use of hallucinogens can also lead to panic, depression, violent reactions, "bad trips" (flashbacks or false perceptions), and brain damage. PCP can be added to marijuana and smoked or swallowed in tablet form. Actually a horse tranquilizer, PCP has a bad effect on people, creating irrational and sometimes violent behavior.

LSD is swallowed as a tablet (a "hit") or in liquid form dropped with an eyedropper onto a small piece of paper ("blotter"). It causes people to hear unspoken voices and see nonexistent visions. LSD also produces panic, nausea, and emotional trauma. Users can experience a "bad trip" which can reappear days or even months after use.

Mescaline and Ecstasy ("X")are swallowed in tablet form. Magic mushrooms ("shrooms") are usually dried and eaten whole or made into tea. The effects of all three drugs are similar to those of LSD, but the hallucinations are less vivid. Users feel that they have endless amounts of energy. Ecstasy is a dangerous drug.

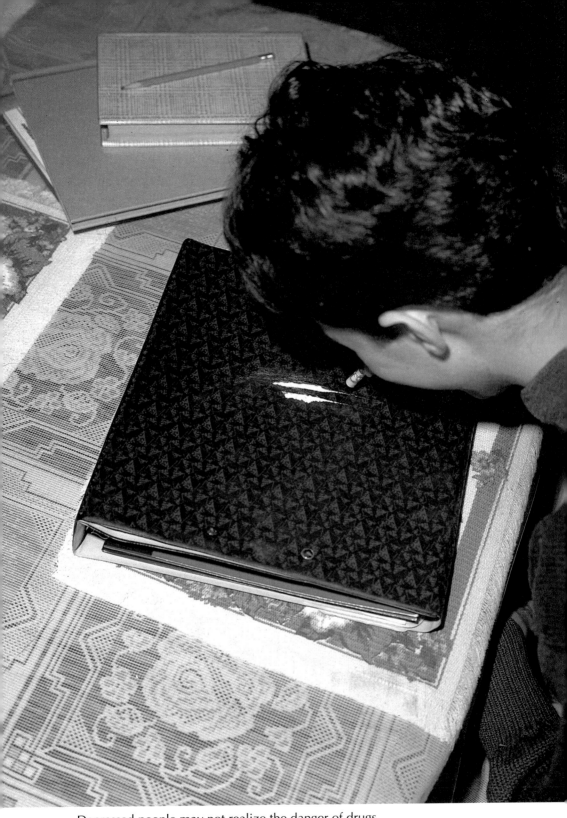

Depressed people may not realize the danger of drugs.

26 | Users experience increased body temperature, dehydration, nausea, sweating, and rapid heartbeat. They also can experience "bad trips," depression, increased anxiety, and paranoia.

Peyote comes from cactus plants. It causes hallucinations. It can be chewed, dried, smoked, or blended into a drink. Some Native Americans have used peyote in religious rituals to enter trance-like states and communicate with spirits.

Inhalants. Inhalants include glue, gasoline, paint thinner, cleaning fluids, and aerosol sprays. The fumes from these substances are either breathed in directly from their container or poured into a bag and held over the face. This type of inhaling is called huffing. Young people inhale these fumes for the quick head rush they get. Inhaling can cause headaches, dizziness, convulsions, brain damage, and heart failure.

At a Glance

The chart on pages 27 and 28 shows the kinds of drugs and substances teens use and abuse when they feel depressed. It also shows the expected effect of each drug, and its risks and dangers.

Drug/ Substance	Type of Drug	Expected Effects	Dangers
Alcohol	Depressant	Relaxation and reduced anxiety	Impairment of physical and mental functions, liver and kidney disease, black-outs, alcoholism
Opiates (heroin, China White, Special K, barbiturates, sedatives, codeine, opium)	Depressant	Extreme happiness, dreaminess, relief from pain	Nausea, impaired physical and mental ability, convulsions, HIV/AIDS (if injected), coma, death
Ampheta-mines (white crosses, speed, crystal meth, ice, crank)	Stimulant	Increased arousal, alertness, energy	Restlessness, headaches, loss of sense of reality
Cocaine/ Crack	Stimulant	Extreme happiness, dreaminess, relief from pain	Nausea, impaired physical and mental ability, convulsions, HIV/AIDS (if injected), coma, death
Caffeine	Stimulant	Increased attention, quicker reactions, greater alertness	Insomnia, irregular heartbeat, restlessness, increased blood pressure

Drug/ Substance	Type of Drug	Expected Effects	Dangers
Nicotine (cigarettes, cigars, pipe and chewing tobacco, snuff)	Stimulant	Increased relaxation, greater alertness	Heart disease, cancer, respiratory problems, decreased circulation
Marijuana	Hallucinogen	Relaxation, pleasant feeling, seeing things differently	Distorted senses, nausea, impairment of learning and judgement
LSD	Hallucinogen	Hallucinations, increased energy, false sense of understanding or increased knowledge	Panic, nausea, emotional trauma, "bad trips," flashbacks, loss of sense of reality, brain damage
PCP (angel dust), peyote, mescaline, magic mushrooms (psylocibin)	Hallucinogen	Hallucinations, increased energy, false sense of understanding or increased knowledge	Panic, nausea, emotional trauma, "bad trips," flashbacks, loss of sense of reality, brain damage
Ecstasy	Hallucinogen	Feeling good, increased energy, sense of confidence, relaxation, reduced anxiety, heightened senses	Panic, nausea, sweating, increased body temperature, rapid heartbeat, moodiness, insomnia, "bad trips", depression, anxiety, paranoia
Glue, gasoline, paint thinner, cleaning fluids, propellants	Inhalant	Quick head-rush, extreme happiness, dreaminess	Headache, dizziness, disorientation, confusion, convulsions, brain damage, heart failure

Drugs and Depression

Using illegal drugs puts a temporary Band-Aid on problems. The reasons for the depression are never addressed, and the symptoms return time and time again, worse each time. The crash after the high often leaves users far more anxious or depressed than they were to begin with. Other problems begin to pile up such as health risks, endangering yourself and others through unsafe behavior, and difficulties with family members, friends, and the police. When an addict needs a "fix," classes, assignments, homework, friends, and family become unimportant. Any kind of responsibility takes a back seat.

Abusing drugs as a method of coping with depression is never a solution. Only by seeking professional help, and through the positive support of friends and family can the causes and symptoms of depression be addressed and relieved.

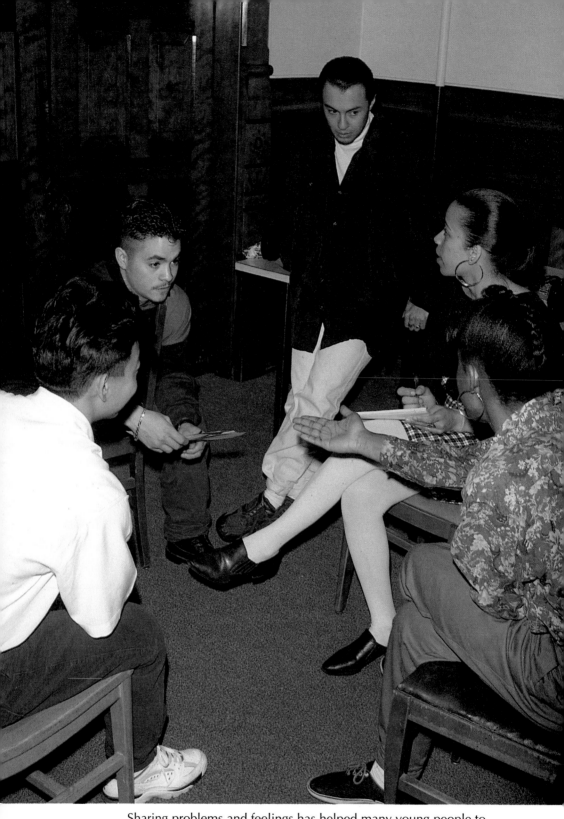

Sharing problems and feelings has helped many young people to overcome their fears and take responsibility for their lives.

CHAPTER 3

Getting the Message

SOS, or Starting Over Self-assured, is a
fellowship group designed especially for
teenagers who have had trouble with
drugs and depression. Once a week, 10 to
16 young people meet in the cafeteria of
Neil Armstrong High. The atmosphere is
relaxed and informal. Usually someone
brings chips or pizza. Members also use
the soda machine in the hallway. Everyone has agreed to follow certain rules,
including no putdowns or swearing.
Sometimes that is not easy. Another
agreement is that everything said is to remain confidential. "When I start to cry,
and sometimes I just can't help it," says
Judd, "I don't want anyone spreading it all
around school."

"I guess we've talked about everything there is to talk about," Larkin says. "We discuss things we can't tell our parents and don't want to tell our school counselors. I trust the kids in the group. We feel close to one another because of the crummy things that have happened. We don't pass judgment because we're all in the same boat and we hurt. A lot."

"The important thing," Judd says, "is that we're all learning that fighting our depression is also fighting fear. I know that sounds strange coming from someone who is over six feet tall and a halfback, but believe me, I have a lot of fears. I need validation...approval, like anyone else. Because of the way I look, people tend to forget that."

Tough Times

Stephen and Christy are also members of SOS. They live at a treatment center. Stephen is 17 years old, a recovering alcoholic, and is often overwhelmed by severe depression. Part of his depression is caused by feelings of guilt. When he was 15, he became a drug pusher to support his drinking habit. As a child, alcohol was readily available in his home. Stephen's parents were alcoholics. They did nothing to discourage him from drinking; they often shared their beer with him.

"I feel bad about all the kids I turned onto drugs," Stephen says. "I pushed junk like 'reds,' 'pink hearts,' and 'cross tops.' Those are names for speed, which keeps a person hyper all the time. I sold a lot of drugs to seventh-graders because kids that age are naive. Eighth-graders seem smarter, and ninth-graders make choices either to use dope or not to use it. I also sold to gang members.

"My mom left my dad because he knocked her around. She also left me. My dad didn't care about me. He said he wished I'd never been born. He said that a lot. My dad finally dumped me off onto my grandfather. Granddad was really good to me. I quit drinking when I was with him. Then he became sick and died of pneumonia.

"For a while, I lived in a foster home. I started drinking again because the other kids there drank. We hung out in the park and had wild times. I realize what I experienced as a child had a lot to do with my drinking problem. I know, too, that I have to be responsible for myself. I like going to the SOS meetings, and I've joined Alcoholics Anonymous, too."

34   Stephen is learning how to deal with his feelings. "Through counseling, I am getting help for severe depression," Stephen says. "I've learned some important things: (1) I *can't* change the past. (2) I *can* change myself. (3) With determination and outside help, I can help to fix myself.

"For a long time I hated my life, and drinking was the only thing that helped. Nothing seemed important. Family, friends, school—nothing mattered. I felt like I was floating between pain and boredom. Sometimes I was jittery and jumpy. I know now that drugs are not a solution. Instead of helping, everything gets worse. A person can't outrun depression. When I was drinking, I had this feeling of being lost, abandoned. I've done a lot of bad stuff, and I regret it. I try not to look back, to condemn and torment myself. Trust me, I know that a person can change. I know, too, that it isn't easy."

More Tough Times

Christy says that even when she was nine years old she often felt depressed. Her mom drank, and her stepfather abused her mentally and sexually. She was always fighting with her brothers and sisters. She was often locked in her room. Christy felt

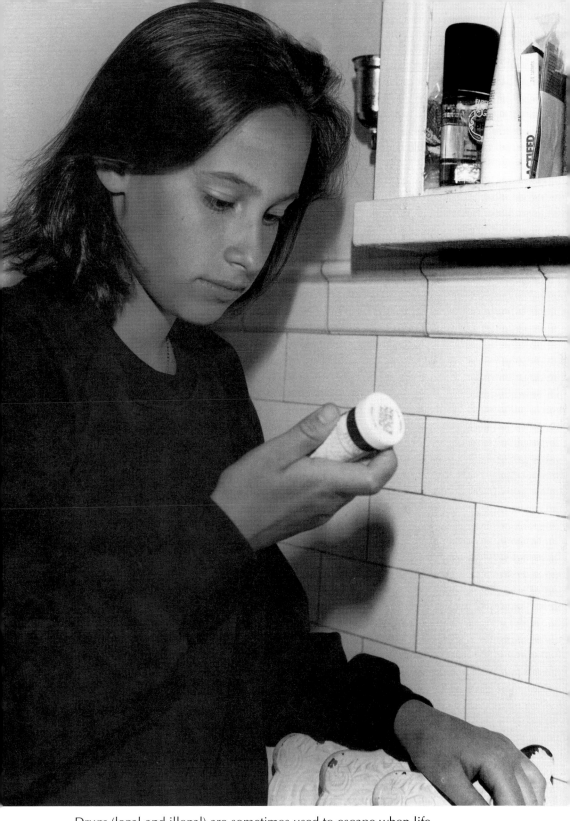

Drugs (legal and illegal) are sometimes used to escape when life seems unbearable.

36 confused and scared most of the time. There never seemed to be anyone for her to talk to when she needed help.

Christy discovered that drinking cough syrup made her forget her problems. Once in a while, she sniffed glue or nail polish remover. Sometimes she sniffed hair spray. She was in the sixth grade when she noticed bottles of pills in the family medicine cabinet. The pills looked harmless. They were pretty colors and looked like tiny Easter eggs. She found out that she was more relaxed if she swallowed a few pills before going to school. One day the school notified Christy's parents that their daughter was sleeping through most of her classes. There was a big family fight. Christy continued to sneak prescription pills, but she was more careful. She "saved up" what she took, and when she felt overwhelmed by life she took them all at once. For a while they made her feel better. Then things got worse. She often picked fights at school, and she started smoking on the playground.

In junior high, people offered Christy marijuana and other street drugs. She used them every chance she got. Her depression became more severe, and her behavior became more bizarre. "I stabbed a friend," Christy says. "The school, the kid's parents, and my parents hushed it up."

Christy goes on to say, "I think my problems started with my home life. My parents were always loaded, and my little brothers and sisters needed attention that I was too young to provide. I have spent a lot of my life being angry and hating myself. Being on drugs and often being depressed causes a kind of isolation. Right now, with the help of a counselor and taking the right amount of medication, I'm learning to work through my problems. I am beginning to know there are some good things about me...I'm a good listener and I am a truthful person. I don't lie. I am also a good worker. I am trying to learn how to have friends. It used to embarrass me when someone complimented me, but now I like it when someone says I've got a great smile. I know there will come a time to shut the door on all the trash and misery that I have lived with. The best thing, after all the bad stuff, is knowing I'm not crazy. I never was, although I admit that I was certainly mixed up. It's scary to think you might be insane. I know there's a lot of wonderful things out there in the world. I want my share."

38 | ## *Consequences of Depression*

Instead of reaching out for help, sometimes teenagers turn their pain inward and do things that make them hurt even more. These are some of the destructive behaviors that may accompany depression:

Eating Disorders. Depression is a major cause of eating disorders such as anorexia nervosa (self-starvation), bulimia (bingeing on large quantities of food and purging), and compulsive eating (bingeing without purging). Obsessing over body image and food can give the depressed person a false sense of control over himself.

Drug and Alcohol Addiction. Some teens turn to drugs and alcohol to hide from reality. When they are stoned, it is easy to forget about the concerns of day-to-day life. Drugs and alcohol can be used to try to make pain and discomfort go away.

Self-Mutilation. Cutting, hitting, or burning their bodies are other ways teens cope with depression. This usually happens when a person's emotional pain is so great that inflicting physical pain on himself or herself creates a release and a diversion. The physical pain of self-mutilation tends to numb the mental pain, or at least, that is how the person rationalizes it.

Suicide. Of the millions of Americans |
who experience serious depression every
year, about 500,000 are teenagers who
try to kill themselves. Suicide attempts
can often be a cry for help. When people
feel it is impossible to commucicate ver-
bally about what is bothering them, or
when they can think of no more options,
suicide can seem like the only way out.

Elaine and Ho-Kim

*Elaine and Ho-Kim met at a rock concert.
Elaine was high on coke and Ho-Kim was
smoking weed. They became friends and
started hanging out and skipping school. They
thought it was fun to be high all the time.*

*"When I was high," said Elaine, "I didn't
have to think of the problems I had at home."*

*"Yah," said Ho-Kim, "with Ma always
drunk and yelling at me all the time, it just
felt better to be out of it."*

*Elaine and Ho-Kim were depressed because
of things going on in their homes. They both
used drugs to ease the pain. Eventually they
were both suspended from school. But they
were lucky. The vice-principal told them about
free counseling and said that once they got
cleaned up, he would clear their school record.*

*Thanks to Mr. Campbell, Elaine and Ho-
Kim had a chance to recover.*

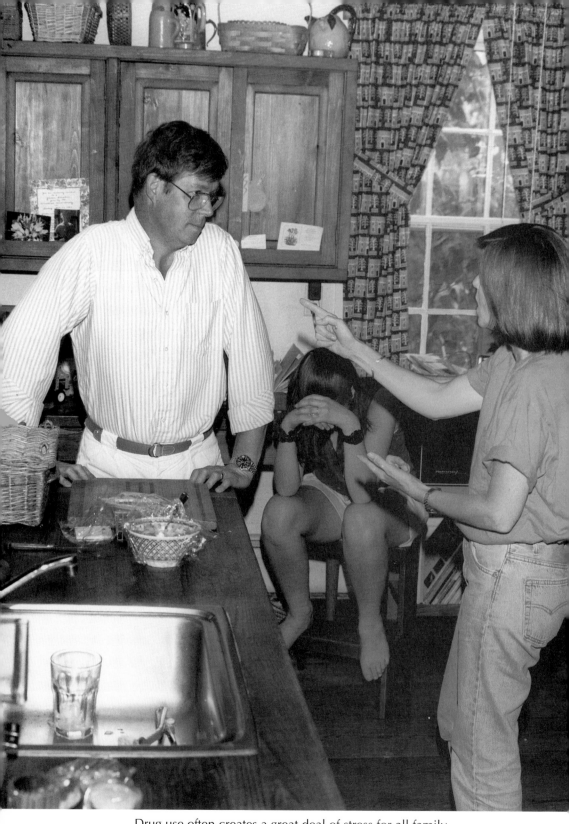

Drug use often creates a great deal of stress for all family members.

CHAPTER 4

Facing the Truth

Severe stress threatens many of today's households because of drug use. Low self-worth tends to be part of the package if one lives in a home where feelings are not valued and needs are not met. Family members become neglected. Language is abusive. Expressions of affection are neither said nor shown. Rules and expectations change from one day to the next. Life becomes confusing. Family members have to guess what is normal. For some, the abnormal is normal. That may mean sexual abuse, physical abuse, or dad's and mom's heavy drinking. Family members may turn to overeating, anorexia, bulimia, or drugs as a way to escape their problems. Depression only worsens. It may become impossible to function normally on a daily basis.

42 The only way to resolve feelings of depression is to get problems into the open. That means talking to someone. The someone can be a parent, a sibling, another relative, a friend, a teacher, a counselor, or a mental health professional. Joining a support group can be helpful. These organizations first enable members to identify their feelings. They are encouraged to express themselves. They talk about problems such as appropriate and inappropriate behavior. They learn to relate to others. They learn how to cope with their stress. They learn to heal their wounds.

Groups

These organizations have names like Challenge, Crossroads, Miracles, Gain, and New Beginnings. Many use the word *anonymous* in their name; for example, **DA** or Depression Anonymous. Topics of discussion may be substance abuse, enrolling in a new school, adjusting to a new stepparent, or any number of other hurdles that can arise during the teen years.

Many special programs are patterned after Alcoholics Anonymous, or **AA**, started 50 years ago by a man named Bill who knew that people needed to talk out their pain. Support groups encourage understanding, prevention, and intervention.

Many Student Assistance Programs have been established. Most elementary, junior high, and high schools offer voluntary classes on drugs and depression.

Miracles

Mary Nelms is a group facilitator, which means that she guides group discussions. She facilitates a class about depression. It is called Miracles. The purpose of the group is to talk about what plunges a person into the depths of depression. Everyone is frank and truthful. All stories are kept confidential. D., a junior in high school, readily admits that drug dependence is a major problem in her life. "My main focus is to party-party," she says. "Like most drug users, I seek the high, also called 'catching a bus'. I have developed an increased drug tolerance. I know this because it takes more stuff to get happy. My priorities at school are the same except I have new friends and they are important because we can share drugs. When I dope, I'm fearless and turned on, but when I come down I have a lot of guilt and crummy depression. I wish I could change."

44   The positive side of D.'s story is that she admits she is doing something destructive. With help, understanding, and encouragement from her peers at the weekly Miracle meetings, she may soon be able to make more positive changes in her life-style.

Like D., we have all done something we wish we had done differently. The truth is, it's not possible to reach back in time and unsay mean words or undo rotten behavior. We can, however, learn to make better choices. It is a myth that people cannot change or be rehabilitated until they hit rock bottom. They may decide that the only answer left is an about-face. With determination, great effort, definite goals, positive thinking, and—above all—being kind to oneself, people, including D., can meet the challenge.

Miracle's guidelines for overcoming problems:

- Express feelings
- Practice restraint
- Make conscious choices
- Practice problem-solving
- Develop listening skills
- Develop communication skills
- Don't live in the past, live today
- Develop an understanding of self and others

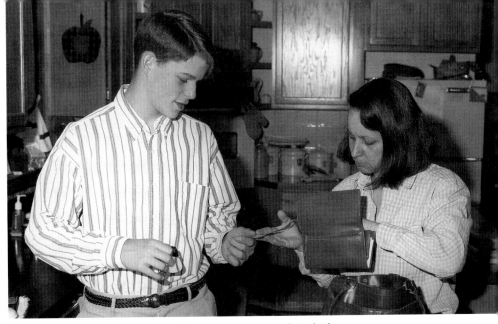
Children need limits. Parents who can't say no to their kids are not doing them any favors.

- Learn what situations cause feelings of depression
- Know that without positive help you will be a casualty.

Getting Well
Students in Ms. Nelms's class have learned that the progression of drug dependency is predictable and that depression is part of the picture. This runaway course consists of use, abuse, and dependency. Members also know that the relapse rate is high. Setbacks are often part of the disease. Therefore, recovering drug addicts need routine and a positive outlook. They also need patient and understanding friends and family. Depression, one of the most common mental disorders, is also the most responsive to therapy.

46   The kids who have joined Miracles know they have to get involved in things they would not usually find interesting. Exercise programs, sports, and music may be some of these activities. The key is to stick to a choice, whether it is swimming or learning to tap dance. Determination can be a lifeline. It can lead to self-confidence, self-control, and self-esteem.

Enabling

The noun "enabler" and the verb "enabling" have fairly new meanings in our vocabulary. Enablers accept or even encourage undesirable behavior. Usually they do this unwittingly. Sometimes they believe things will get better. They ignore an illegal act to make excuses for bad conduct. In that way, they send a message that unacceptable behavior is okay. They are enabling because they allow the drunk, junky, pusher, liar, thief, or sexually irresponsible person to continue reckless behavior.

The Easy Way

As a small child, Evan had tantrums. His parents quieted him with cookies and candy—it was easier that way. In high school, Evan demanded pocket money, a

car, and even a credit card. His parents
complied—it was easier that way. One
morning the principal telephoned Evan's
parents. He told them their son was sit-
ting in his office—drunk. A Breathalyzer
test proved it. "No way," Evan's father
said. "The kid may have taken a sip out
of a bottle in the cupboard, but that's it."
Because the police had been called, Evan
was given a fine, which his parents paid—
it was easier that way.

Evan's parents were enablers. They
turned their heads when their son had
problems. They did nothing to discourage
or correct his negative behavior. They ig-
nored his angry outbursts by saying it was
only normal teen behavior. It was easier
that way.

School counselors, teachers, and the
principal gave up on Evan's parents long
ago. They have never given up on Evan.
They still hope that he will turn his life
around. Who knows? He just may. The
decision is his.

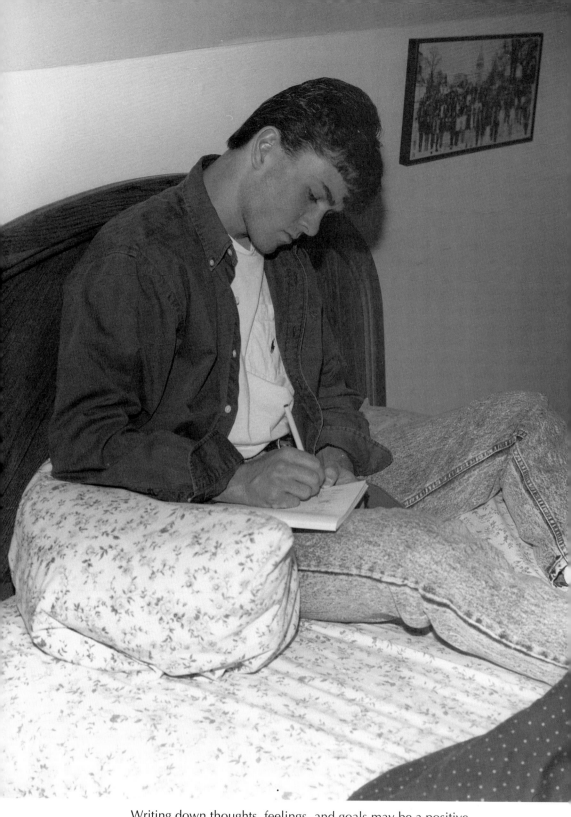

Writing down thoughts, feelings, and goals may be a positive way to understand your needs and find healthy ways to meet those needs.

CHAPTER 5

Working It Out

*D*epressive disorders make you feel exhausted, worthless, helpless, and hopeless. Such negative thoughts and feelings make some people feel like giving up. It is important to realize that these thoughts are part of the depression, and *not* part of who you are as a person. Negative thinking fades as treatment for depression begins to take effect. There are many kinds of treatments and support systems for depression.

Help from Family and Friends
The most natural support system for many people is family and friends. Talking to someone you know and trust is a good first step. Sometimes, however, as much as others want to help you, people who

50 have never experienced depression may not fully understand its effect. It may be helpful to share some information about how your family and friends can best help you get through this difficult time.

Family and friends can help a depressed person get appropriate treatment. This may involve encouraging the person to stay with a therapy or antidepressant medication until the depression lifts, or to seek different therapists or antidepressant treatments if no improvement occurs. It can be helpful for a family member or friend to go with the depressed person to the doctor. He or she may also help keep track of whether the depressed person is taking the medication properly.

Family and friends can also offer emotional support. This involves understanding, patience, affection, and encouragement. When talking with the depressed person, listen carefully. Don't criticize his or her negative feelings. Instead, point out some realities and offer hope. Try to engage the depressed person in activities such as going for walks or going to the movies. Family members and friends should be gently insistent if their invitations are refused. Encourage participation in activities that once gave the depressed person

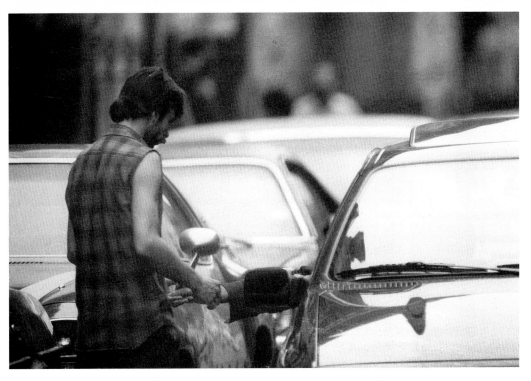

Drug users need to get drugs constantly in order to satisfy their "habit."

pleasure, such as a particular hobby or religious or cultural activity. But do not push the depressed person to take on too much too soon. Too many demands can increase feelings of failure.

Finally, never accuse the depressed person of faking illness or of laziness. And don't expect him or her to just "snap out of it." Reassure the person that with time and help, he or she will feel better.

Therapy

Sometimes talking to family members and friends is not enough. You may need to move beyond your immediate circle to some of the resources provided by your community. Schools usually employ psy-

52 | chologists or social workers. If you don't know how to find the psychologist or social worker at school, ask a teacher whom you trust. Also, a school social worker can refer you to an outside therapist if you prefer. If your family has health insurance, you can find a qualified therapist/ counselor through your insurance company. If you do pursue therapy, it helps to know what kind of therapists are available.

- Psychologists and licensed social workers have a master's degree or Ph.D. in psychology and have completed many years of training. They can conduct one-on-one or group therapy.
- Psychiatrists are trained psychologists who are also medical doctors. They also can do one-on-one or group therapy. They are authorized to prescribe antidepressant medicine.
- Many forms and styles of therapies are used effectively to help depressed individuals, including some short-term (10-20 weeks) therapies.
- "Talking," or interpersonal therapies, help depressed individuals focus on their problems with personal relationships that both cause their depression

and make it worse. Talking therapies help individuals understand and re-solve their problems through a verbal give-and-take with the therapist.

- Behavioral therapies help depressed individuals to change their negative styles of thinking and behaving. Behavioral therapists guide individuals to learn how to obtain greater satis-faction and reward through their own actions, and how to "unlearn" certain behavior patterns that con-tribute to their depression.

Choosing an appropriate therapist and a kind of therapy that feels right for you is a huge step toward feeling better about yourself and your life.

Medication
If medication is part of your therapy, be sure to take it exactly as directed. Pay close attention to how the medicine is affecting you. Talk to your psychiatrist or therapist about how you feel. Remember that medication does not take the place of therapy—they work together.

Helping Yourself
Remember that while getting professional help, you can also do many things to help

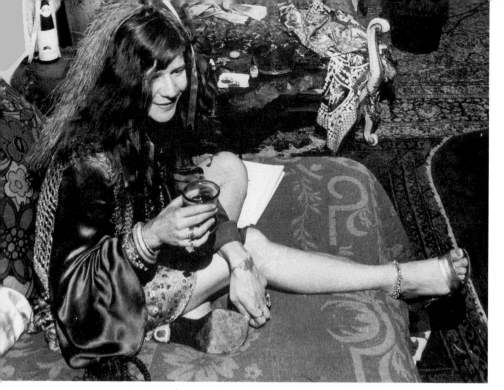

Janis Joplin was America's number one female rock singer when she died of a drug overdose in 1970.

yourself. This is important because it can give you a feeling of self-satisfaction and control over your own life. Here are some things that you can do for yourself:

- Do not expect too much from yourself too soon.
- Do not set difficult goals for yourself.
- Break large tasks into smaller ones, and do only what you can.
- Try to be with other people; it's better than being alone.
- Participate in activities that may make you feel better.
- Don't be upset if your mood is not greatly improved right away.

• Do not make major decisions such
as dropping out of school, changing
jobs, or breaking off a relationship
without talking with someone who
knows you well. It is best to wait
until the depression has lifted before
making big decisions.

Recovery from Addiction

Depressed people who then become addicted to drugs have a harder time recovering, but recovery is possible. Recovery
may take many weeks or months, but it
will save your life.

If you or someone you know is strug-
gling with a drug problem and is ready to
do something about it, the most important thing to do is find help. If for some
reason you don't feel comfortable approach-
ing someone you know, check the yellow
pages for listings under Drug Abuse Counseling and Social Service Organizations.
It is important to get help quickly. Many
treatments are available for successful recovery from drug addiction. They include:

• Inpatient treatment—a live-in hospi-
tal or clinic that keeps you safe while
you are withdrawing from drugs.
Many clinics are free.

56

- Twelve-Step programs—free meetings held by other recovering drug abusers. The Twelve Steps are principles of spiritual self-discovery. By "working" the steps, you develop a support system.
- Therapy—one-on-one or group meetings run by a therapist. Meetings with a therapist or trained professional in the mental health field can be as successful for recovery from drug addiction as they are for recovery from depression.

Saying No to Drugs

It sounds so easy, doesn't it? Just say no! But the truth is that saying no takes a lot of will power and courage. When you hurt, taking drugs may seem like a good way to get away from the pain. When your friends experiment with drugs, it's hard to feel left out. With drug pushers right in your neighborhood, it's hard not to be tempted. If alcohol or pills are in your home, what's to stop you?

If you care about yourself and those around you, take pride in having the strength to say no. It shows strength of character, determination, and self-respect. You can avoid temptation and situations

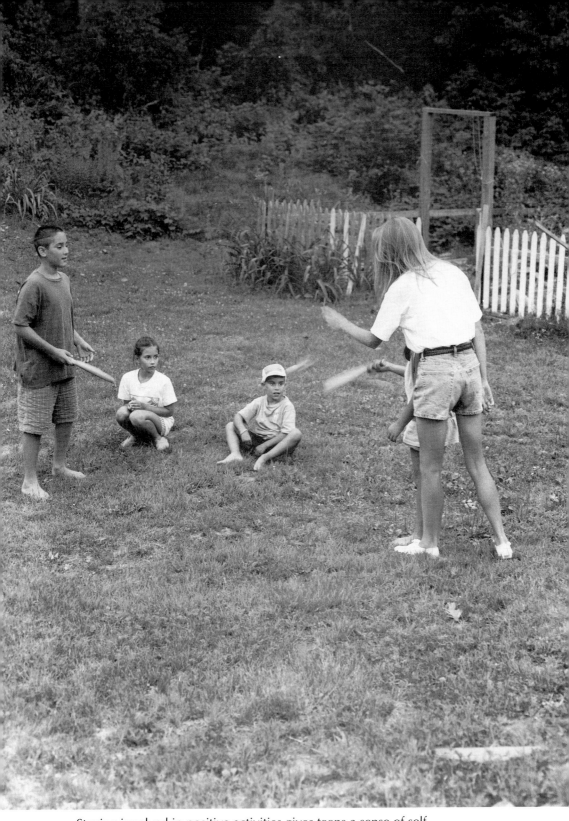

Staying involved in positive activities gives teens a sense of self-worth and satisfaction.

58 where drugs are present. There are also ways to say no to drugs without feeling embarrassed.

- Keep yourself occupied with activities you enjoy.
- Choose your friends carefully.
- Educate yourself. Read magazines and articles about the reality of drugs and their abuse. Know what drugs and alcohol do to your body and to your mind. Forget about the Hollywood and television industry of drinking, smoking, doping, and drugging. It doesn't tell the whole story. Fast lives lead to fast deaths.
- If you are experiencing feelings of depression or anxiety, remember that drug and alcohol abuse makes those feelings worse.
- Steer clear of drug dealers and people who associate with them.
- If you cannot avoid someone offering you drugs, and you feel embarrassed to just say no, make up an excuse. Say you have a medical condition that makes it dangerous for you to take the drug. Or say that your father is a police officer, and he'd spot you high a mile away.

Glossary

AIDS (acquired immunodeficiency syndrome) An incurable viral disease.

anorexia nervosa An eating disorder characterized by fasting to the point of starvation.

bipolar depression Having two extreme behaviors.

bulimia An eating disorder characterized by binges followed by induced vomiting.

compulsion Strong urge to act contrary to one's will.

enabler A person who supports another person's unacceptable behavior.

euphoria Exaggerated sensation of well-being.

insomnia Chronic inability to sleep; sleeplessness.

unipolar Single process of disturbed state of mind.

Where to Go for Help

General Help for Drugs and Depression
Consult the Yellow Pages of the phone book under: Alcoholics Anonymous, Alcoholism, Chemical Dependency, Counselors, Drug Abuse, Mental Health Services, Social Workers, and Therapists.

Hotlines

Anxiety/Panic Hotline
(800) 647-2642

National Youth Crisis Hotline
(800) 448-4663

Suicide Prevention Hotline
(800) 227-8922

Mental Health Crisis Hotline
(800) 222-8220

United States:

Al-Anon or Alateen
P.O. Box 862, Midtown Station
New York, NY 10018-0862
(800) 356-9996

Covenant House
A safe haven for kids who are hurting. You can call to talk from anywhere in the world.
(800) 999-9999
http://www.covenanthouse.org/kid/kid.htm

Narcotics Anonymous
P.O. Box 9999
Van Nuys, CA 94109
(818) 773-9999

National Alliance for the Mentally Ill
200 North Glebe Road,
Suite 1015
Arlington, VA 22203-3754
(800) 950-NAMI

National Depressive and Manic-Depressive Associations
730 North Franklin Street, #501
Chicago, IL 60610
(800) 826-3632
http://www.ndmda.org

National Foundation for Depressive Illness, Inc.
P.O. Box 2257
New York, NY 10116
(800) 248-4344
http://www.depression.org

Obsessive Compulsive Foundation
P.O. Box 70
Milford, CT 06460
(203) 878-5669

Phobics Anonymous
P.O. Box 1180
Palm Springs, CA 92263

Canada:

Al-Anon
1771 Avenue Road
P. O. Box 54533
North York, Toronto, Ontario
  M5M 4N5
(416) 410-3809
http://www.al-anon.org

Alcoholics Anonymous
AA Central Office
807 Main Street, West Unit B
Hamilton, Ontario L8S 1A2
(905) 522-8399
http://www.aa.org

Canadian Mental Health Association
2160 Yonge Street, 3rd Floor

Toronto, Ontario M4S 2Z3
(416) 484-7750
http://www.cmha.ca

Covenant House Toronto
20 Gerrard Street East
Toronto, Ontario M5B 2P3
(416) 598-4898
http://www.covenanthouse.org

Covenant House Vancouver
575 Drake Street
Vancouver, British Columbia
  V6B 4K8
(604) 685-7474
http://www.covenanthouse.org

Narcotics Anonymous
(416) 691-9519
http://www.members.better.
  net/toronto_na/na.htm

The Stress Doc
(202) 232-8662
http://www.stressdoc.com/teen
  _depression_series.htm

Web Sites

Anxiety Disorders
http://www.nimh.nih.gov/ publicat.anxiety.htm

Federation of Families for Children's Mental Health
http://www.ffcmh.org/info.htm

New York University Department of Psychiatry
"Online Depression Screening Test"
http://www.med.nyu.edu/ Psych/screens/depres.html

Plain Talk About Depression
http://www.nimh.nih.gov/ publicat/ptdep.htm

For Further Reading

Arrick, Fran. *Tunnel Vision*. New York: Bradbury Press, 1980.

Ayer, Eleanor H. *Depression*. New York: The Rosen Publishing Group, Inc., 1997.

Ball, Jacqueline A. *Everything You Need to Know About Drug Abuse*, rev. ed. New York: The Rosen Publishing Group, Inc., 1994.

Clayton, Dr. Lawrence, and Carter, Sharon. *Coping with Depression*, rev. ed. New York: The Rosen Publishing Group, Inc., 1992.

Cunningham, Julia Woolfolk. *Come to the Edge*. Philadelphia: Pantheon Books, 1977.

Edwards, Gabrielle I. *Coping with Drug Abuse*, rev. ed. New York: The Rosen Publishing Group, Inc., 1990.

Grosshandler, Janet. *Coping with Alcohol Abuse*. New York: The Rosen Publishing Group, Inc., 1990.

Hughes, Dean. *Switching Tracks*. New York: Atheneum Publishers, 1982.

Lee, Jordan. *Coping with Anxiety and Panic Attacks*. New York: The Rosen Publishing Group, Inc., 1997.

National Institute of Mental Health, "Plain Talk About Depression." NIH Publication No. 94-3561, U.S. Department of Health and Human Services, http://www.nimh.nih.gov/public/ptdep.htm

Schleifer, Jay. *Everything You Need to Know About Teen Suicide*, rev. ed. New York: The Rosen Publishing Group, Inc., 1993.

Sherrow, Victoria. *Mental Illness*. San Diego, CA: Lucent Books, Inc., 1996.

Silverstein, Virginia, and Alvin Silverstein. *Diseases and People: Depression*. Springfield, NJ: Enslow Publishers, Inc., 1997.

Index

About the Author

Beth Wilkinson has taught elementary school, high school reading and literature, and special education. Professional affiliations include membership in professional organizations and groups interested in literature, music, adult literacy, the young child, antiques, and art. Ms. Wilkinson lives in Laramie, Wyoming.

Photo Credits

Cover photo by Dick Smolinski; p. 21 © Associated Press; pp. 51, 54 © Wide World Photos; all other photos by Stuart Rabinowitz.